Table of Contents:

Introduction:

All praises to the mighty Yahweh!!! Thank you for deciding to read this very enlightening book, I would first like to give all praises to the mighty one of ya'akov (Jacob) and the redeemer of Israel, Yahweh the Elohim of Abraham, the Elohim of Isaac and the Elohim of Yisrael!!! He is the creator and the only savior of yisrael and the world! Yahweh is the holy name of who many just call god, or the lord, Jehovah etc. the almighty's name is Yahweh! And I also would like to honor and respect my teachers: The Late Mowreh Elesha yisrael, the man of Elohim and prophet of Yahweh, my teacher from the House of Yisrael of Cincinnati OH, and Mowreh Ishiyah Ben Yisrael of the House of Yisrael of Raleigh north Carolina, these great men have taught me the laws, statutes and judgments of the most high and if it weren't for their diligent instruction I would be amidst the congregation of the dead today!

I also must acknowledge my elders in the field of natural and holistic health, my first teacher in holistic health the late Elijah(Greg)Taylor, and his wife erin taylor, Nemmsaiu Amen-Sebek, ND.,_Dr, Sebi, Dr. afrika and many more who've I've learned so much from whether personally or by reading and listening to you.

Also I would like us to remember our ancestors who were stolen from their dwelling places in west Akubulan and forced into a life of cruel bondage, who found the need to keep living and not give up and never stopped telling their seed the truth of who we are, if it weren't for our ancestors we would not know a thing! HaleluYAH!!!

Message to the Sick Man
By Mowreh IshYAH Mal'ak YisraEL

To eat that food you eat is this good for you? Do you know where it came from, do you even know where you come from. This is the trick they've played on us for so long, to give us death to the point where we think that life is wrong.

In the book of Isaiah the 55 chapter the 1-3vs YAHWEH asked us why are we laboring for that which is not bread and eating that which does not satisfy us? The black man and woman in the western hemisphere has been sold a bag of snake oil, we take on everyone else's way of life and end up serving them harder than they do for themselves, We give our all into looking and acting like the one's who've oppressed us but never consider ourselves, (Is 1:1-3) The Most High Said to the Children of Yisrael do not learn the ways of the Heathen, and choose none of the ways of the wicked. We the Children of YisraEL have gone absolutely against this warning. The Black man and woman in the USA are the descendants of the True Hebrew Israelites, and we prove this by reading the book of Deut 28:15-68, you'll notice that we are the only people that have been cut off from our true identity, and never returned to our homeland, and have had great terrors and plunders befall us, many nations take control of us and make of us bywords and proverbs, in addition we are the sickest people on the planet and you'll see in Deut 28, that these and more is what YAHWEH said would happen to us.

Therefore I write this book to focus on my people but if anyone is sick you will be healed if you follow the guidelines given in this book. I did not write this book, I did not come up with these ideas, and I am simply explaining the words of the Almighty to you when it comes to health. My training is in Natural and Holistic Health, and there are many books in the earth that attempt to tell you how to become healthy but I've never seen a book that told you like it is, just how YAHWEH said it, an this is what I'm attempting to do with this book, If you want to Really eat to live then The Most High's Natural Health plan will show you how.

You'll notice in this book we do not once speak about the New Testament, this is because YAHWEH never spoke in the New Testament and never gave anyone in the New Testament to be anyone special for the salvation of the Black man or the world. To show why we will not ever speak of this character in the book, if you look in Matt. 15:16-20, and I Corinthians 10:25 here you'll see JC and Paul, condoning the eating of anything! This is troublesome because it is that philosophy that has many of our people disease ridden today. Also you'll see JC stating in Matt 5:39, to resist not evil, again by accepting harm to your body is very unhealthy, also, Luke 14:26, JC tells us to hate our community, and if you hate your community but love your enemy as JC stated in Matt. 5:44, then you'll ignore me and listen to *the Wizard of OZ* who tells you it's ok to eat unnatural YAH forbidden food. Actually the reason why we are sick today is greatly because of the worship of Christ, you'll also see In the book of I Timothy 5:23 that Paul tells you to not drink water, but wine for your ailments, and water is the far most important thing you can put in your body! So the New testament nor the Christ in it does not give you sound health advice, lastly Mark 11:12-13, shows us that JC didn't know the seasons, so how could he teach us the right way to eat?????

If we are to become healthy, we must start by freeing ourselves, For some you might have to free your body first, you might have to get your health together before you free your mind, and then you can free your spirit, the order of how one must free themselves will vary from person to person, For me I had to Free my spirit first, I had to liberate my spirit from the oppressor's society, that enslaved me, my family, people, and ancestors for nearly 400 years. Once I saw that YAHWEH was the truth, I was able to free my body, and now that My spirit and body were free, My own mind is free, and when your mind is free you learn how to depend on the Almighty and not ever worry about man who's breath is in his nostrils. Although some might need a free mind before they free there spirit, as I said the order is different for everyone. Yet one thing I know for sure, As long as someone has their foot on your neck, you won't be able to see everything that is good for you unless the pressure from that foot is loosened, therefore my people with this book I'm attempting to show you how to loosen that pressure, our health is completely under our control, we can choose good or choose wrong ways to live, and our health is the first thing that will be impacted from either choice. So I urge you to consider the instruction given in this small book to show you The Most High's Natural Health Plan!

The Most High's Natural Health Plan

1. Why Should I Eat?

The Creator gave order to everything he made and there is an order to eating. If we go outside that order we'll experience disorder, this will cause a maelstrom of dis-ease in our bodies. YAHWEH did give us a reason why we should eat and not be an airatiarian as some people profess. Look at Deut 8:3 *And he humbled thee, and suffered thee to hunger, and fed thee with manna, which thou knowest not, neither did thy fathers know; that he might make thee know that man doth not live by bread only, but by every word that proceedeth out of the mouth of YAHWEH doth man live.*
Job 23:12 *Neither have I gone back from the commandment of his lips; I have esteemed the words of his mouth more than my necessary food.*
Ecc.10:17 *Blessed art thou, O land, when thy king is the son of nobles, and thy princes eat in due season, for strength, and not for drunkenness!*

I Kings 19:6-8 And he looked, and, behold, there was a cake baken on the coals, and a cruse of water at his head. And he did eat and drink, and laid him down again.

7And the angel of YAHWEH came again the second time, and touched him, and said, Arise and eat; because the journey is too great for thee.

8And he arose, and did eat and drink, and went in the strength of that meat forty days and forty nights unto Horeb the mount of Elohim.

Also read Ps 107:4-9 They wandered in the wilderness in a solitary way; they found no city to dwell in.

5Hungry and thirsty, their soul fainted in them.

6Then they cried unto YAHWEH in their trouble, and he delivered them out of their distresses.

7And he led them forth by the right way, that they might go to a city of habitation.

8Oh that men would praise YAHWEH for his goodness, and for his wonderful works to the children of men!

9For he satisfieth the longing soul, and filleth the hungry soul with goodness.

To be hungry essentially means to feel or be weak, and the Almighty shows in his book that we eat for strength, not for drunkenness, and for ultimate strength all we need is the word of YAHWEH and for physical strength he gave us food. Therefore is any type of food good? Did YAHWEH make everything and say that he gave us everything for food or did he give us specific creations for food?

2. What should I Eat?

It is very important we let not man tell us what is good or perfect for us to eat, because man did not make man, man does not know about everything in our bodies, but the Creator does Ps 103: 14- *For he knoweth our frame; he remembereth that we are dust.* Therefore our best source to find out what we should eat should come from the Almighty himself.

Also a note in diet here, YAHWEH does not like us to be fat e.g. Eglon a Moabite king was so fat when he got stabbed dirt came out of his body, Ps 17:8-10 we see Wicked oppressors are Fat.... *Keep me as the apple of the eye, hide me under the shadow of thy wings,*
From the wicked that oppress me, from my deadly enemies, who compass me about.
They are enclosed in their own fat: with their mouth they speak proudly. And Ps 119:69-*70 The proud have forged a lie against me: but I will keep thy precepts with my whole heart. Their heart is as fat as grease; but I delight in thy law.*

The Prideful man's heart is as fat as grease! Also when Yisrael was rebellious YAHWEH said Jeshuran waxed fat and kicked- Deut 32:15, Lastly the Almighty made it against the law to eat Fat in Lev. 3:17 *It shall be a perpetual statute for your generations throughout all your dwellings, that ye eat neither fat nor blood.* The Fat he is speaking of is the fat of beast, because we know we can classify the oil from plants, as fat or fatty acid, but this fat YAHWEH is mentioning is the fat of beast.

Therefore the food the Almighty instructs us to eat will not make you fat and I know for a fact that the food YAHWEH instructs you to eat will destroy excess fat. So what should we eat? Well of course we should drink water. Next look at these scriptures and investigate what YAHWEH gave us to eat: Gen 1:11-12, 29, Lev. 11, Lev 19:19, Deut 22:9, Deut 20:19-20. As we can see the scriptures instruct us to only plant non-mingled vegetation, eat non-fattening meats, fruits, vegetables, and clean meats. And we are not to eat any fattening foods, or raw meats. So where does this leave us in a society that sells mostly mingled (Hybrid) seedless foods?

It leaves us in a place esp. the Black man and woman in America, in which we must return to the ways of our ancestors and grandparents, who've always planted their own food- Jer 6:16 *Thus saith YAHWEH, Stand ye in the ways, and see, and ask for the old paths, where is the good way, and walk therein, and ye shall find rest for your souls. But they said, We will not walk therein.* And Read Jer. 29:4-7. Yes, YAHWEH did instruct us to seek after the old and good ways and plant gardens.

Hybrid foods are foods that have been genetically modified to grow in conditions, and

varieties not possible in nature. For instance, Egyptians hybrid onions and made garlic, you'll see that the children of YisraEL just like today loved that garlic- Numbers 11:4-6 *And the mix multitude that was among them fell a lusting: and the children of Israel also wept again, and said, Who shall give us flesh to eat? We remember the fish, which we did eat in Egypt freely; the cucumbers, and the melons, and the leeks, and the onions, and the garlick:*
But now our soul is dried away: there is nothing at all, beside this manna, before our eyes.
Now major food distributers thrive from producing and selling GMO and hybrid foods. The foods that are GMO whether plant or animal, are very questionable for consumption. Most GMO foods esp. plants are Hybrids according to YAH. This means 99.9% of everything you buy in your grocery store is useless according to the Creator: Deut 22:9 *Thou shalt not sow thy vineyard with divers seeds: lest the fruit of thy seed which thou hast sown, and the fruit of thy vineyard, be defiled.*

If you want to be healed it is very simple eat the food YAHWEH gave us to eat, life and death can not abide together if you fill your spirit, soul, and heart with life, then death must be evicted. Ps 103:5 *Who satisfieth thy mouth with good things; so that thy youth is renewed like the eagle's.*

<u>Here is a list of Natural foods</u>
Amaranth greens - same as Callaoo, a variety of Spinach

Avocado

Asparagus

Bell Peppers

Burro Banana

Chayote (Mexican Squash)

Cucumber

Dandelion greens

Garbanzo beans (chick peas)-optional

Izote – cactus flower/ cactus leaf- grows naturally in California

Jicama

Kale

Lettuce (all, except Iceberg)

Mustard greens

Nopales – Mexican Cactus

Okra

Olives

Onions

Purple Potato

Red Skin Potato

Poke salad -greens

Sea Vegetables (wakame/dulse/arame/hijiki/nori)

Squash

Spinach (use sparingly)

String beans

Tomato – cherry and plum only

Tomatillo

Turnip greens

Zucchini

Lentils (Preferably Red Lentils)

FRUITS - " no canned or seedless fruits".

Apples

Bananas – the smallest one or the Burro/mid-size (original banana)

Berries – all varieties- Elderberries in any form – no cranberries

Cantaloupe

Cherries

Currants

Dates

Figs

Grapes -seeded

Limes (key limes preferred with seeds)

Mango

Melons -seeded

Orange (Seville or sour preferred, difficult to find)

Papayas

Peaches

Pears

Plums

Prunes

Raisins -seeded

Soft Jelly Coconuts

Soursops –Latin or West Indian markets)

Sugar apples (chermoya)

ALL NATURAL HERBAL TEAS
There are more Herbal teas that are natural this list is not exclusive you must to your own research on everything you eat.
Alvaca

Anise

Chamomile

Cloves

Fennel

Ginger

Lemon grass

Red Raspberry

Sea Moss Tea

SPICES & SEASONINGS

Mild Flavors

Basil

Bay leaf

Cilantro

Dill

Marjoram

Oregano

Sweet Basil

Tarragon

Thyme

Pungent & Spicy Flavors

Achiote

Cayenne

Cumin

Coriander

Onion Powder

Sage

Salty Flavors

Pure Sea Salt

Powdered Granulated Seaweed

(Kelp/Dulce/Nori – has "sea taste")

Sweet Flavors

100% Pure Maple Syrup – Grade B recommended

Maple "Sugar" (from dried maple syrup)

Date "Sugar" (from dried dates)

100% Pure Agave Syrup – (from cactus)

NUTS & SEEDS -(includes Nut & Seed Butters)

Raw Almonds and Almond butter

Raw Sesame Seeds

Raw Sesame "Tahini" Butter

Walnuts/Hazelnut
Raw Brazil Nuts

GRAINS

Amaranth

Black Rice

Kamut

Quinoa

Rye

Spell

Tef

Wild Rice

Barley

Millet
Emor

Hybrid(English Definition) The offspring of two animals or plants of different breeds, varieties, species, or genera, especially as produced through man manipulation for specific genetic characteristics.

What does YAHWEH Say about mixing plants and animals?

Read Leviticus 19:19 *Ye shall keep my statutes. Thou shalt not let thy cattle gender with a diverse kind: thou shalt not sow thy field with mingled seed: neither shall a garment mingled of linen and woollen come upon thee...*

Read Deut. 22:9 *Thou shalt not sow thy vineyard with divers seeds: lest the fruit of thy seed, which thou hast sown, and the fruit of thy vineyard, be defiled.*

There are a couple of key words that need to be addressed in both of these scriptures:

- Divers/Mingled- 3610 Strong's Concordance- Kilayim- Sense of separation two heterogeneities- divers seeds(-e kinds) mingled (seeds)

- Kind- Strong's Concordance 4327- Miym (meen) to portion out; a sort i.e. species-kind.

YAH does not want his people to produce cattle and plants that are of different kinds, which are of different species. We can look at how various animals and plants mix in nature, and they are able to mix because they are of the same kind. Although a mule would be an unlawful cattle in YAH'S kingdom as would be the mixing of Grapes and apples.

Oranges, Kale, Collard greens, wheat, and more are all hybrids but not mixed from different kinds. True hybrids according to YAH are two different kinds. Read Lev. 19:19 *"thou shalt not sow thy field with mingled seed...."* And Gen 1:11 YAH said he made everything after its own kind having a seed. YAH also let us know he made all the fish, the beast, the fowls, and the creeping things after their own kind.

YAH said in Jer. 29 :4-7 that we should plant vineyards and gardens. It is imperative for us to know what type of vegetation is lawful to plant and eat.

1. If we eat Oranges, Broccoli, and Collard Greens are we going against YAH'S law?
    a. No, YAH gave us clear instructions of what we can eat and can not even among the plant kingdom: Read Gen 1:29-30 *And Elohim said, Behold, I have given you every herb bearing seed, which is upon the face of all the earth, and every tree, in the which is the fruit of a tree yielding seed; to you it shall be for meat. And to every beast of the earth, and to every fowl*

of the air, and to every thing that creepeth upon the earth, wherein there is life, I have given every green herb for meat: and it was so.

If we encounter fruit that does not have seed and it should, this is not natural and not what the Creator gave us to eat. Although Oranges, Broccoli, and Collard Greens are among common hybrids according to today's standards they are hybrids of their own kind. See Chart below:

Citrus Kind	Cabbage Kind
Oranges	Broccoli
Lemons	Brussels sprouts
Limes	Kale
Mandarin	Mustard Greens
Tangerine	Bok Choy
Pomello	Cabbage

All the above-mentioned plants are cultivated, and to be cultivated it is a hybrid in order to produce a desired variety. Nevertheless they are not mixed of anything but it's own kind.

2. Why is it important to know what is a hybrid according to YAH'S law?
   a. This is important because YAH requires us to bring the first fruits Lev. 23:10-21, and he said the

mingling of seed would cause it to be defiled Deut. 22:9

Therefore if we plant vegetation that is not after it's own kind, then it will be defiled and unfit for Holy offerings and unfit for our own land.

What food shouldn't we Eat?
Any thing with Soy, white Wheat, White, or Brown rice, White potatoes.

Mushrooms- If we again look at Gen 1:11-12 *And Elohim said, Let the earth bring forth grass, the herb yielding seed, and the fruit tree yielding fruit after his kind, whose seed is in itself, upon the earth: and it was so.*
And the earth brought forth grass, and herb yielding seed after his kind, and the tree yielding fruit, whose seed was in itself, after his kind: and Elohim saw that it was good.
We see the Almighty made three types of vegetation: Grass(Sprouts, sprouting) Herbs (Plants), Trees. Now let's go verse 29 *And God said, Behold, I have given you every herb bearing seed, which is upon the face of all the earth, and every tree, in the which is the fruit of a tree yielding seed; to you it shall be for meat.* We see YAHWEH did not mention that he gave us grass to eat for meat. Proverbs 30:5-6 States do not add to

YAHWEH'S word lest he reprove thee and thou be found a liar. Therefore if we understand that mold, mildew, and other fungi are not creeping things, nor fish, beast, or fowl, nor do they have a seed inside itself, we can deduce that mushrooms and it's fungal relatives, are the sprouting that Elohim made and he did not tell us he gave it to us for food. So, should we eat mushrooms? NO!!

3. When Should I Eat?

Proverbs 23:1-7
When thou sittest to eat with a ruler, consider diligently what is before thee:
And put a knife to thy throat, if thou be a man given to appetite.
Be not desirous of his dainties: for they are deceitful meat.
Labour not to be rich: cease from thine own wisdom.
Wilt thou set thine eyes upon that which is not? for riches certainly make themselves wings; they fly away as an eagle toward heaven.
Eat thou not the bread of him that hath an evil eye, neither desire thou his dainty meats:
For as he thinketh in his heart, so is he: Eat and drink, saith he to thee; but his heart is not with thee.

In this passage we see wisdom explaining to be careful what you eat when sitting before powerful people,, just because they've bidded you to a feast does not mean we should eat their food. The word states put a knife to thy throat if you are a man given to appetite also we see in prov 21:17 One that loves pleaser, wine, and oil, shall not be a rich man but be poor. And loads of money is not what makes you rich, for how happy are you if you're a gabillonare and laid up in a hospice bed because you've loved pleasure, and gave yourself to appetite. Also Daniel knew of this, this is why we see Daniel in the 1st Chapter refusing the king's meat and requesting vegetables and water.

The body has its ordinance, and we see by Solomon's wisdom there is a season for everything even eating. We have already observed this scripture but let's look at it again for some more understanding

Ecc 10:16-17 *Woe to thee, O land, when thy king is a child, and thy princes eat in the morning! Blessed art thou, O land, when thy king is the son of nobles, and thy princes eat in due season, for strength, and not for drunkenness!*

Ok, now we see that eating a fat breakfast every morning is not prudent! The Almighty wants us to eat for strength. Follow the course of nature in the morning a heavy meal will weigh you down, who wants to be weighed down while they begin their task? Ps 104:22-23 *The sun ariseth, they gather themselves together, and lay them down in their dens. Man goeth forth unto his work and to his labour until the evening.*

We know by midday we've worked up a good appetite, but there is more work to do, therefore, food for strength and not weight is our best option. Foods for Strength include: Kale Salads/wraps, Raw Black Rice bowls, fruit, Moringa Shakes, Sea Veggie wraps. You'll notice all this food can be made uncooked because cooked food will work your body too hard while your trying to work hard.

So now our dinners, they can be our heavier meals, three to four courses, a little baked bread or lightly cooked veggies, (Occasionally something lightly fried in Grape seed oil, or coconut oil. If you follow the order of YAHWEH then you'll eat for strength(Health, Life), and not Drunkenness!(McDonalds, Burger King eating at fast food restaurants). *Proverbs 13: 25 The Righteous eateth to satisfying of his soul: but the belly of the wicked shall want.*

4. <u>Where should I get my food?</u>
I know your saying "Yeah IshYAH I know what your saying is good, but where the Hell am I supposed to get all this food from?!" *When you find out send me an email, imyisrael@gmail.com....* Seriously- Natural food's best market is the earth itself, but many of us do not know the right time to water artificial grass let alone plant our own food. Therefore this is where your decision on lifestyle starts to really play a factor. First you'll start by going to the stores, then you'll find there that it's not so wholesome.

Second you'll look for farmers markets, and see hybrid farmers, and hybrid food!

Now you'll start thinking about your own backyard, now if this was your first thought, the 5k you spent on these other options, you could've had a nice garden IshYAH!!.... I'm sorry back to the you the reader... We can go to the various natural food markets, and you'll find they'll have some of what we need but if you don't make it yourself you probably won't see it on your plate... The Almighty let his people know in Jer. 29:4-7 to plant their own gardens. You'll also see that Daniel had to get food from the slave master, but he asked for Vegetables. For my people are destroyed for lack of knowledge. If we do not seek to learn how to grow our own food and make our own meals then we will never be FREE!!! YAHWEH said in Isa 10:20 that the children of YisraEL shall no longer Stay(Lean, Cling, depend) upon him that smote them, but shall stay upon YAHWEH, the Holy one of YisraEL in Truth!

Where we get our food from should be our own backyard gardens, in house pots, sprouting jars, raised gardens, community-co-op gardens etc. If we care about our children then we wouldn't allow them to eat the food from the schools we shouldn't be sending them to.
When it comes to where should meat eaters eat... The proverbs state in Prov. 27:23, that you should know the condition of your flocks. If you don't then how will you know if these beast are fed grain or pig brain??? And the overwhelming evidence, that many meat manufactures are

mishandling their animals should make you at least consider where you're getting your flesh from. Also the Law in Leviticus 17:15-16 *And every soul that eateth that which died of itself, or that which was torn with beasts, whether it be one of your own country, or a stranger, he shall both wash his clothes, and bathe himself in water, and be unclean until the even: then shall he be clean. But if he wash them not, nor bathe his flesh; then he shall bear his iniquity.*

Also read Deut 14: 21. We are not to eat anything that dieth of it self, and many beast that people eat have died of themselves in the meat factories.

All fast food restaurants ignore the separation of clean(non toxic) and Unclean(Toxic) animals. They'll put pizza's in ovens glossed over with swine juice from pepperoni, sausage, and bacon lovers pizza. You'll find French fries and fried shrimp in the same grease, bloody beef all over the counters worms crawling on cutting boards from sliced ham... and so on. My parents used to say when we asked; "where are we eating tonight" they would say "At the Brown's."

<u>How Should I Eat?</u>

Ok, So we've discussed; why, what, when, and where to eat, but How do we actually do this? Do we eat this food Raw or cooked? Fresh or preserved? What is the best way?

Raw or Cooked?

If you are a meat eater then your food should be cooked very well done all the time. The various times we see the children of YisraEL eating meat the meat was always grilled very well done. For those that believe every meal should be raw, I say that the Creator disagrees. Although a majority fresh food diet is the best way to eat. The book of Psalms in the 104th verse states: He Causeth the grass to grow for the cattle and the herb of the field is for the service of man that he may bring forth food out of the earth. Also look at verse 15, YAHWEH did not explicitly say only eat food raw or eat food cooked, but if you also look at EzekiEL 47:12, YAHWEH let's us know that the fruit of the tree is for food and the leaf is for medicine. There are little to no fruits that cannot be eaten raw. The best way to eat fruit and leaves are raw.

Yet sometimes these foods are used cooked. Herbs are cooked oftentimes when medicines are made, and leaves and fruit are still lively if you allow them to soften in hot water. If we consider that a plant is alive and so are we therefore if you're in a pot boiling for 45min-1hr, then you'll die, and if you douse yourself in oil and sauté yourself for minutes on end you'll die. If you put yourself in a oven for 30min-2hrs, you'll die, but if you go into a steamer you'll live and if you relax yourself in a Jacuzzi that is very hot you'll live. Well plants are the same, fry them, bake them, or boil them, you'll most likely kill them. Dead food is not beneficial to our bodies, nor for nutrition or for healing.

Now let's not be too sorrowful, bread is still good if we bake it, how do I know this? "Because the word of YAHWEH let's me know." I I Kings 19:6-8 we see that Elijah was given Baked or Grilled Bread to sustain him for forty days and nights. Now if there was an absolute evil with eating cooked food why would the Almighty give EliYAH, cooked bread? Also in Leviticus the 2nd chapter the Almighty described to us that meal (grain) offerings can be oven baked, pan baked, or fried. And the priests were to eat it, and we know that YAHWEH didn't want his priest unhealthy.

We must also consider the various ways we can manipulate grain. The book of Deut 24:6 let's us know that a millstone is very important to a man's life, and why is that? Because this millstone is what we use to grind grain look at Isa 47:2; if the only nutritious way to eat grain was to snap it right off the stem then YAHWEH would not make a law concerning an instrument used to grind grain seeds.

Therefore, How do we eat? Mostly fresh is how we should eat. Cooked food should be occasionally, if we notice in the scriptures our people had cookouts and they were big family reunion type of parties and you can see when we had them by reading Leviticus chapter 23, and Deut. 14: 22-28

The Secret to perfect Health is to do the whole duty of man- Fear YAHWEH and keep his Commandments!

NATURAL AND FRESH FOOD RECIPES BY YAEL S. YISRAEL

Raw Kale Wrap

2-4 Servings   30-60
minutes prep time

1 bushel of raw fresh kale
chopped green onions
1 chopped avocado
1 chopped tomato
sea salt
1 lime
sprouted wraps/pita bread
raw dressing/chickpea humus

Place fresh kale in a large bowl or a clean kitchen sink with a stopper on the drain. Gradually, squeeze the juice from the lime onto the kale and add a few pinches of sea salt. Use clean hands to massage the kale until it begins to feel tender. Add the avocado, tomato, and green onions.

Continue to massage and mix the ingredients until the kale mixture is very tender. At this point, the kale leaves will seem smaller and more condense then before. Spread your favorite raw dressing or chickpea humus onto a Raw seaweed wrap (Nori). Add the raw kale mixture and fold the wrap.

Recipe#8 Ruby Red Quinoa Soup

8-10 servings
30 minutes prep time

1-2 chopped tomatoes
1-1/2 c fine string beans
1c spinach
1 lg. chopped yellow onion
1c red quinoa
2 tomatoes puree
cumin, cayenne, sea salt
rinse quinoa, warm tomato puree and 2-1/2 c water until slightly soupy consistency, add veggies, and cook down. Add quinoa. Stir, Simmer 20 minutes.

Raw Super GOOD Burger

BURGER:
1c walnuts (dry/soaked)
handful of raisins
1/4c sundried tomatoes
3T dulse flakes
3T Hemp seed protein powder
3T nutritional yeast
1/4c olive oil

SEASONING:
Onion powder
Curry
Cumin
Sea salt
Cayenne pepper

DRESSING:
coconut wraps (cut in half)
avocado
sliced onions
kale
special sauce/tahini/ketchup/mustard/etc.

Process ingredients in Vita mix until a firm pate is formed. Add seasoning to mixture. Blend well. Dress burger and enjoy.

RAW 'THE BOMB' LASAGNA

SAUCE:
1 ½c Sundried tomatoes
Olive oil

CHEESE/MEAT:
4 handfuls of Raw Nuts (Pecans or Cashews, Walnuts, etc.)
½ lime Juice Squeezed
Sea Salt

NOODLE:
3 Cucumbers or Zucchini, Eggplant, etc.
Lightly Salted

VEGETABLE:
4 cups Spinach or Kale

TOPPING:
1 Avocado
1/4c Raw chopped Walnuts

First, thinly slice the Noodle vertically. Blend the Sauce to a smooth thick cream. Next, blend the Cheese/Meat to a chunky, fluffy cream. In a large dish layer ingredients as follows: Noodles, lightly salt, Cheese/Meat, Vegetable, Sauce, Repeat. Add topping. Chill or Serve immediately.

Raw-licious' Fruit Pie

CRUST:
2 cups Nuts (hazelnuts, almonds, walnuts, , Brazilian)
1 cup of pitted Dates (apricots, figs, raisins, etc.)
Salt

SAUCE:
2 cups Fruit (sorted, washed, cut/seeded/pitted)
½ lime juice squeezed
1 cup of pitted Dates (soak)

FRUIT:
2 cups of fruit (blueberry, strawberry, cherries, etc.)

Blend the crust in food processor until crumbly. Place crust in pie dish and mold the crust and chill in freezer 15 minutes. Blend the sauce in blender until a smooth liquid. Place fruit in large bowl and mix in the sauce. Stir well. Place the mixture inside crust. Chill 1 hour in the fridge. Serve and Enjoy!

Really Good Spelt/Amaranth Quick Bread

2 ½ c Spelt Flour
½ c Amaranth Granules
1tsp. Baking Powder
½ tsp. Baking Soda
1tsp. sea salt

    1/3 c Grape seed Oil
    1c Almond Milk
    1/4c water

Combine dry & wet ingredients; mix well. Preheat 350 degrees. Lightly oil bread pan. Cook 30-45 min. Yields 6-12 servings.

Delicious Quick Barley Biscuits

- 2 cups Barley flour
- 1 tbsp baking powder
- 1/2 tsp salt
- 4 tbsp Coconut oil
- ¾ cup Homemade Almond milk

Preparation:

Pre-heat the oven to 450 degrees.

Put all the dry ingredients into a bowl. Using a fork, blend the oil into the dry ingredients until the mixture breaks down into fine particles.
- Add the Almond milk and stir until the particles cling together. Turn out onto a floured

bread board or countertop and knead for 1 to 2 minutes or until the dough is smooth. Add more flour as needed if the dough is sticky

References

Holy Bible; King James Version.
Food List: drsebiproducts.com

The House of YisraEL of Cincinnati is a Hebrew
Biblical and Cultural Center and our mission is to bring
YisraEL the so-called Black Man and Woman in
America back to the Creator who's name is YAHWEH!
If you would like more information about the House of
YisraEL please visit this website:

www.worldgatheringyisrael.org

May YAHWEH bless thee and keep thee
May YAHWEH lift up his countenance unto thee and be
gracious unto thee
May YAHWEH make his face shine upon thee and give
the Peace! HaleluYAH

www.ingramcontent.com/pod-product-compliance
Lightning Source LLC
Chambersburg PA
CBHW070241290526
45789CB00004B/1715